Stroke Savvy

How to Avoid and Bounce Back from a Stroke in 20 Steps

By

Dwight W. Gagne

DISCLAIMER

Table Contents

Introduction

Stroke is a grave medical disorder that annually affects millions of individuals worldwide. It happens when a portion of the brain loses its blood supply, which results in the death of brain cells and irreversible harm to the brain's ability to function. Physical, mental, and emotional impairments brought on by strokes can have an impact on the survivors' and their families' quality of life.

The good news is that if we identify a stroke early on, we can treat and prevent it. The risk of stroke is increased by several variables, including obesity, sedentary lifestyle, smoking, alcohol consumption, high blood pressure, high blood sugar, high cholesterol, and cardiac issues. You can lower your risk of stroke and enhance your general health by managing these variables and forming healthy habits.

It's critical to take quick action and get medical help as soon as you suspect that you or someone you love is having a stroke. Your chances of surviving and recovering are better the earlier you begin therapy. There are efficient therapies that can lessen the damage caused by stroke and restore blood flow to the brain. These medications, however, have a limited window of opportunity and need to be administered within a few hours after the onset of symptoms.

It can take a while to fully recover from a stroke, so support, patience, and perseverance are essential. You may have a variety of impairments, including weakness, numbness, paralysis, speech difficulties, vision problems, memory issues, emotional difficulties, and behavioral changes, depending on the location and degree of the stroke. It might take a variety of therapies for you to restore your abilities and adjust to your new circumstances. It can also be necessary for you to modify your surroundings and way of life to enhance your well-being and avoid having another stroke.

You will discover more about stroke in this book, including its definition, causes, symptoms, signs, prevention, treatment options, and recovery strategies. Along with helpful hints and counsel, you will discover how to manage your risk factors, identify and react to a stroke, deal with the psychological, emotional, and physical aftereffects of a stroke, and lead a happy life following a stroke. The purpose of this book is to give you practical advice and information to help you avoid, survive, and recover from a stroke.

Step 1: Control your blood pressure

One of the most crucial things you can do to avoid a stroke and other health issues is to control your blood pressure. The disease known as high blood pressure, or hypertension, occurs when the blood force on the walls of the arteries is very high. This may harm blood vessels and the organs they supply, including the heart, kidneys, and brain.

Several factors, including genetics, age, gender, ethnicity, and lifestyle, can influence blood pressure. You have some control over some of these things, but not over others. By changing your diet, exercise routine, lifestyle, and prescription drugs, you can reduce your blood pressure.

The following advice can help you manage your blood pressure:

Consume a balanced diet. Your blood pressure can be lowered by eating a diet high in fruits, vegetables, healthy grains, lean meats, and low-fat dairy products. Steer clear of foods heavy in added **sugars, cholesterol**, saturated fat, and salt. The DASH (Dietary Approaches to Stop Hypertension) diet is an excellent illustration of a healthy diet. Exercise regularly. Engaging in physical activity helps enhance blood circulation and strengthen your heart. Additionally, it can aid in weight loss, which lowers blood pressure. Try to get in at least 150 minutes a week of moderate-to-intense aerobic activity, such as swimming, cycling, or brisk walking. 2. To strengthen your bones and muscles, try doing strength training activities twice a week.

Give up smoking. Smoking can raise blood pressure and cause blood vessel damage. It may also raise your chance of lung cancer, heart attacks, and strokes. Give off smoking as soon as you can. You can get help quitting using a variety of tools and therapies, including gums, lozenges, inhalers, sprays, patches, counseling, and medicine. 3. Set an alcohol limit. Excessive alcohol use can damage your heart, liver, and brain, in addition to increasing your blood pressure. Additionally, it may conflict with several blood pressure-lowering drugs. If you consume alcohol, do so sparingly. For women, that means no more than one drink per day, and for men, no more than two drinks per day. Twelve ounces of beer, five ounces of wine, or 1.5 ounces of liquor make up one drink.

Control your tension. Stress can impact your mood, sleep quality, and overall health, in addition to raising your blood pressure. It may also cause you to start engaging in harmful habits like binge eating, smoking, or drinking. Try to recognize and stay away from the stressors in your life to manage your stress. Additionally, you can engage in relaxation exercises like yoga, massage, meditation, and deep breathing. Getting adequate sleep, hanging out with loved ones, reading, listening to music, and engaging in hobbies are further strategies for lowering stress.

Keep an eye on your blood pressure. Monitoring your blood pressure will enable you to identify any changes and modify your treatment plan as necessary. You can take your blood pressure using a digital blood pressure monitor at home, in a clinic, drugstore, or doctor's office. **Blood pressure** should not be higher than 120/80 mm Hg. See your doctor about the best course of action if your blood pressure is greater than that. Consume your prescription drug. Your doctor may recommend medication to help decrease your blood pressure if lifestyle modifications are insufficient. Angiotensin-converting enzyme (ACE) inhibitors, calcium channel blockers, diuretics, angiotensin II receptor blockers (ARBs), and other medications are among the several kinds of blood pressure medications. Your doctor will select the medication that best matches you, taking into account each one's unique advantages and disadvantages. When taking medication, adhere to your doctor's recommendations; do not stop taking it or alter its dosage without first talking to your physician.

In addition to preventing a stroke, controlling your blood pressure can enhance your general health and well-being. You can maintain a healthy blood pressure level by lowering it with the help of these tips. Always monitor your blood pressure, and if you have any questions or concerns, don't hesitate to speak with your doctor.

Step 2: Control your blood sugar

Your body uses glucose, also known as blood sugar, as its primary energy source. On the other hand, extreme blood sugar levels can lead to major health issues like diabetes, heart disease, and nerve damage. Consequently, it's critical to maintain healthy blood sugar levels by controlling them.

A variety of factors can influence your blood sugar levels, including the foods you consume, the amount of activity you get, your level of stress, and the drugs you take. We'll go over some of the best natural blood sugar-lowering strategies in this article to help you avoid problems. Among these techniques are:

Consuming a diet low in processed carbohydrates and added sugars and high in fiber, protein, and healthy fats

Getting frequent exercise and maintaining an active lifestyle

Keeping hydrated and consuming adequate water

Controlling your stress levels and engaging in relaxation methods

Taking your prescription drugs as indicated and routinely checking your blood sugar levels; speaking with your doctor before changing your lifestyle or course of treatment

You can lower your chance of acquiring diabetes and other chronic diseases and improve your blood sugar control by using the advice in this article. Recall that maintaining blood sugar control benefits not only your physical well-being but also your emotional state, vitality, and standard of living.

Step 3: Control your cholesterol

Your blood contains a waxy material called cholesterol, which is necessary for the production of hormones, vitamin D, and bile acids, among other body processes. On the other hand, excessive cholesterol can be dangerous since it can clog your arteries and raise your risk of heart disease and stroke. Low-density lipoprotein (LDL) and high-density lipoprotein (HDL) are the two primary forms of cholesterol. People often refer to LDL as "bad" cholesterol because it transports cholesterol from the liver to the cells and can lead to artery plaque development. People often refer to HDL as "good" cholesterol because it helps prevent plaque from forming in the arteries and transports cholesterol from cells back to the liver.

A wide range of factors can influence your cholesterol levels, including your genetics, age, gender, nutrition, way of life, and health issues. While you have no control over some of these factors, you can influence others by making healthy decisions. The following are some strategies for lowering your cholesterol: Consume a well-balanced diet rich in fiber, fruits, vegetables, whole grains, healthy fats, and low in trans and saturated fats. Your LDL cholesterol can be raised by trans and saturated fats, while your HDL cholesterol can be raised and your LDL cholesterol lowered by fiber, fruits, vegetables, whole grains, and healthy fats. Foods that are healthy for your cholesterol include avocado, olive oil, salmon, berries, legumes, nuts, and seeds.

Strive for a healthy weight and engage in regular exercise. Engaging in physical activity can help improve your blood pressure, blood sugar, and general health by raising your HDL cholesterol and lowering your LDL cholesterol. Aim for two or more days of muscle-strengthening exercises per week in addition to at least 150 minutes of moderate-intensity or 75 minutes of vigorous-intensity aerobic exercise, or a mix of the two. Obesity and excess weight can raise LDL cholesterol, decrease HDL cholesterol, and raise the risk of several health issues. Your cholesterol levels can be improved, and your risk of heart disease and stroke can be decreased by losing weight.
Give up smoking and drink in moderation. Smoking raises your risk of heart disease and stroke, lowers HDL cholesterol, and damages blood vessels. Giving up smoking can enhance both

your general health and your HDL cholesterol level. In addition to raising your blood pressure, triglycerides, and calories, alcohol can also elevate your HDL cholesterol, which can increase your risk of heart disease and stroke. If you do consume alcohol, make sure to do it in moderation—that is, no more than one drink for women and two for men every day.

If your doctor has prescribed medication, take it. Medication may be necessary to lower your LDL cholesterol and avoid issues if diet and lifestyle modifications are insufficient to control your cholesterol levels. A variety of drugs, including fibrates, niacin, cholesterol absorption inhibitors, bile acid sequestrants, and statins, can decrease your cholesterol. Based on your medical history, risk factors, and cholesterol levels, your doctor will recommend the best course of action for you. Adhere to your physician's advice and take your prescriptions on time.

Maintaining a healthy cholesterol level is crucial for both your general health and your heart health. You can boost your HDL cholesterol, lower your LDL cholesterol, and lessen your risk of heart disease and stroke by implementing these strategies.

Step 4: Quit tobacco use

One of the main avoidable causes of disease and death worldwide is tobacco use. Nicotine, a highly addictive chemical found in tobacco, can make quitting difficult. Smoking increases the chances of lung disease, heart disease, stroke, cancer, and other chronic illnesses, among other health problems.

There are short- and long-term advantages to giving up tobacco use for your health and well-being. Quitting can improve blood circulation, lower blood pressure, minimize the risk of developing certain diseases, and improve your overall quality of life. But quitting can also be difficult and necessitate several attempts and approaches. The following advice will help you stop using tobacco: Decide when to stop and create a plan. Decide on a day in advance to give up smoking and get ready for the hardships that lie ahead. To record your progress and keep track of your accomplishments, you can use an app, a notebook, or a calendar. You can also write down your motivations for wanting to stop and the advantages of doing so. This might support your motivation and goal-focused persistence.

Seek out expert assistance and backing. For help and direction on quitting tobacco usage, speak with your healthcare professional, a counselor, or a quitline coach. They can assist you in selecting behavioral therapy, medicine, or nicotine replacement therapy as the best course of action for you. They can also offer you motivation and emotional support while you're trying to quit. You can also get in touch with other individuals who are attempting to quit or have successfully stopped using tobacco by joining a support group, an online community, or a quit program.

Control your cravings and the symptoms of withdrawal. Cravings and withdrawal symptoms, such as irritation, anxiety, sadness, insomnia, headaches, or weight gain, are common when quitting smoking. These are common and transient indicators that your body is getting used to not having smoke. Various techniques, such as chewing gum, drinking water, breathing deeply, working out, meditating, or diverting your attention with a pastime or activity, can help you manage these symptoms. You can also stay away from situations or people that could tempt you to smoke, like stress, alcohol, and particular people. Celebrate your accomplishments and treat yourself. Giving up tobacco use is a significant accomplishment that needs to be acknowledged and celebrated. Treating yourself to a lunch, movie, book, or present is a great way to celebrate your accomplishments and reward yourself. In addition, you can get compliments and encouraging words from your loved ones and your support system by sharing your accomplishments with them. This might strengthen your resolve to abstain from tobacco use and raise your sense of confidence and self-worth.

One of the best choices you can make for your happiness and health is to stop using tobacco. You can improve your chances of successfully quitting and reap the rewards of living a life free of tobacco by paying attention to these pointers.

Step 5: Limit alcohol use

Consuming alcoholic beverages—such as wine, beer, or liquor—that contain ethanol, a psychoactive chemical that can affect your body and mind, is referred to as alcohol use. Depending on your age, gender, heredity, drinking habits, and other circumstances, alcohol usage can have a variety of negative impacts on your health. Among the potential outcomes are:

Short-term effects: These include altered mood, behavior, judgment, memory, coordination, and reaction time; also, there is a higher chance of violence, accidents, injuries, and alcohol poisoning.

Long-term effects: These include increased risk of several chronic diseases, including cancer, diabetes, hypertension, and stroke, as well as harm to the liver, heart, brain, and other organs.

Alcohol use disorder is characterized by intense alcohol cravings, a loss of self-control over drinking, tolerance to alcohol's effects, and withdrawal symptoms after quitting. Alcohol use disorders need to be treated by professionals and can hurt your social, emotional, and physical health.

On days when adults of legal drinking age consume alcohol, the 2020–2025 Dietary Guidelines for Americans suggest that they should have the option to either abstain entirely or to drink in moderation. The guidelines also recommend a daily limit of no more than two drinks for men and one drink for women. This will help to minimize alcohol use and lower the risk of alcohol-related harm. Your health should drink less than more. Additionally, the Guidelines advise against encouraging anyone who does not currently drink alcohol to start doing so for whatever reason.

These pointers will assist you in reducing your alcohol intake:

Make sure you monitor your alcohol intake and establish a personal limit. To measure and track how much alcohol you consume, you can use an app, a drink diary, or a basic drink chart.

Steer clear of drinking on an empty stomach, as this can enhance the effects and absorption of alcohol. Before and during your drink, eat a well-balanced lunch or snack.

Drink carefully, and mix your alcoholic beverages with non-alcoholic ones like juice, soda, or water. This can assist you in consuming less alcohol and staying hydrated.

Select alcohol-free or low-alcohol beverages, like mocktails, wine spritzers, and light beers. These can assist you in cutting back on calories and booze.

Avoid locations and settings like parties, bars, and social gatherings where you could be tempted to drink more than you intended. Additionally, you may schedule your drinking in advance and choose who you'll drink with, how much you'll drink, and how you'll get home safely.

If you find it difficult to control your alcohol consumption or believe you might have an alcohol use disorder, get advice and assistance from professionals. For help and direction on how to cut back on or stop drinking, speak with your doctor, a counselor, or a guideline coach. You can also get in touch with other individuals who are attempting to quit or have successfully stopped drinking by joining a support group, an online community, or a program for quitting.

Reducing your alcohol intake can improve your health and well-being, both now and in the future. You can minimize your alcohol use and limit your chance of suffering from alcohol-related problems by heeding these guidelines.

Step 6: Maintain a healthy weight

For your general health and well-being, it's critical to maintain a healthy weight. Many chronic conditions, including diabetes, heart disease, and stroke, can be prevented and managed with the support of a healthy weight. Moreover, having a healthy weight can boost your vitality, happiness, and self-worth. You must balance the number of calories you burn through exercise and metabolism with the number of calories you take in from food and beverages to maintain a healthy weight.

Your weight status can be determined by a variety of methods, including body fat percentage, waist circumference, and body mass index (BMI). A popular tool for calculating weight in proportion to height is BMI. It can help you determine if your weight is normal, underweight, overweight, or obese in general. BMI, however, does not take into consideration other variables like age, gender, ethnicity, muscle mass, and bone density that may have an impact on your health. As a result, BMI shouldn't be the exclusive measure of your current weight.

Another measurement that might assist you in determining your current weight and risk of developing health issues is your waist circumference. Excess abdominal fat, which is linked to an increased risk of type 2 diabetes, high blood pressure, high cholesterol, and cardiovascular disease, can be indicated by a wide waist circumference. Men should have a waist circumference of fewer than 40 inches, while women should have a waist circumference of less than 35 inches, according to recommendations from the National Institutes of Health (NIH).

The percentage of fat on your body is known as your body fat percentage. Compared to BMI, or waist circumference, it can provide a more realistic picture of your health and body composition. However, compared to testing BMI or waist circumference, calculating body fat percentage might be more challenging and costly. Diverse techniques exist for determining body fat percentage, including dual-energy X-ray absorptiometry, bioelectrical impedance analysis, skinfold calipers, and underwater weighing. The American Council on Exercise (ACE) provides the following body for both men and women:

Required fat: 2–5% in men, 10–13% in women

Sports people: 6–13% of men and 14–20% of women

14–17% of males and 21-24% of women are fit.

Men's average: 18–24%, women's average: 25–31%

25% or more of males and 32% or more of women are obese.

A balanced diet and regular exercise are essential components of a healthy lifestyle that help you maintain a healthy weight. A balanced diet keeps excess calories, fat, sugar, and salt to a minimum while giving you the nutrients and energy you need for your daily activities. To maintain a healthy weight, you should include a diverse range of foods from several food groups in your balanced diet, such as fruits, vegetables, whole grains, lean protein, low-fat dairy, and healthy fats. Additionally, you ought to consume fewer processed foods, fast food, sweets, and alcoholic drinks. Frequent exercise raises your heart rate, increases sweating and breathing resistance, and strengthens your muscles. Engaging in physical activity can aid in calorie burning, muscle growth, fat loss, and the prevention of weight gain. Physical activity can enhance your blood sugar regulation, bone health, mental health, and cardiovascular health. Adults should engage in muscle-strengthening activities two or more days a week in addition to 150 minutes of moderate-intensity or 75 minutes of vigorous-intensity aerobic activity each week, or a mix of both, according to the 2020–2025 Dietary Guidelines for Americans. Keeping a healthy weight involves more than just the numbers on the scale; it also involves how you feel and carry out your everyday activities. A healthy weight that fits your body and your health objectives can be attained and maintained by eating a balanced diet and getting regular exercise.

Step 7: Exercise regularly

Any physical activity that uses your muscles and causes your body to burn calories is considered exercise. Exercise can improve your mood, energy, and sleep, increase brain function and memory, and prevent or manage chronic diseases, among many other aspects of your health and well-being.

Adults should engage in muscle-strengthening activities two or more days a week in addition to 150 minutes of moderate-intensity or 75 minutes of vigorous-intensity aerobic activity each week, or a mix of both, according to the 2020–2025 Dietary Guidelines for Americans. Among the moderate-intensity aerobic exercises are dancing, swimming, cycling, and brisk walking. A few instances of high-intensity aerobic exercises are sports, running, and jumping rope. Exercises that strengthen muscles include push-ups, weightlifting, and resistance band use.

Finding a physical activity that you enjoy, that works for your skills and goals, and that works with your schedule and finances is essential if you want to exercise regularly. In addition, you must monitor your progress, set clear, attainable goals, and treat yourself when you succeed. To improve your motivation and accountability, you can also look for expert guidance, enroll in a class or club, or locate a partner or group to work out with.

Regular exercise can build your bones and muscles, help you stay strong and prevent falls and injuries, help you maintain a healthy weight, enhance your cardiovascular health, lower your blood pressure and cholesterol, and lessen your risk of diabetes and stroke. Regular exercise can also improve your productivity and creativity, as well as lower your levels of stress, anxiety, and depression. It can also make you feel more confident and good about yourself. One of the best things you can do for your physical and emotional well-being is to exercise daily. You can reap the rewards of a more active and healthy lifestyle by starting and maintaining a regular fitness regimen that suits your needs and using the advice in this article.

Step 8: Get enough sleep

It's critical for your health and well-being to get adequate sleep. In addition to promoting healthy bodily and mental functioning, sleep helps stave off several chronic illnesses like diabetes, heart disease, and stroke. Along with lowering stress and anxiety, sleep can also enhance mood, energy, and memory.

Your age, lifestyle, and health issues will all affect how much sleep you require. However, toddlers and teenagers require more sleep than adults, who typically require 7 to 9 hours of high-quality sleep per night. Maintaining a regular sleep schedule, making your sleeping space cozy and peaceful, and abstaining from drugs like alcohol and caffeine can all help you get enough sleep.

You might be suffering from a sleep condition like insomnia, sleep apnea, or restless legs syndrome if you have problems going or staying asleep or if you feel drowsy or exhausted during the day. Sleep disturbances may necessitate medical treatment and can have an impact on your quality of life, safety, and health. Speak with your doctor, get tested, and start treatment as soon as you suspect you may have a sleep problem.

One of the best things you can do for your physical and emotional well-being is to get enough sleep. You may increase the quantity and quality of your sleep and reap the rewards of a rejuvenating and pleasant night's sleep by using the advice in this article.

Step 9: Manage atrial fibrillation

Heartbeats that are irregular and quick are a common and significant symptom of atrial fibrillation (AF). The risk of heart failure, stroke, and other consequences can be raised by AF. Thus, controlling AF is crucial to preventing or lowering these dangers and enhancing the lives of those who have AF.

The management of AF has four primary objectives:

Maintaining a normal heart rate, which typically falls between 60 and 100 beats per minute, is known as controlling heart rate. This may assist in easing the symptoms of AF, including weariness, palpitations, and chest pain. Medication, such as digoxin, beta-blockers, or calcium channel blockers, as well as pacemakers and ablation procedures, can all be used to control heart rate. Regulating the heart rhythm entails bringing the heartbeat—also known as the sinus rhythm—back to normal and keeping it there. This can lower the risk of heart failure and stroke while also enhancing heart function. Medication, such as antiarrhythmics, cardioversion, or ablation procedures, can all be used to control the heart rhythm.

Keeping a blood clot from developing in the heart and moving to the brain to cause a stroke is known as stroke prevention. This can be accomplished by utilizing drugs like anticoagulants or antiplatelets or by blocking the area of the heart where clots typically develop with a device like a left atrial appendage occluder.

Treating the underlying cause means taking care of conditions like high blood pressure, heart disease, thyroid issues, sleep apnea, or obesity that may cause or exacerbate AF. This can be accomplished by changing one's lifestyle to include things like giving up smoking, drinking less alcohol, maintaining a healthy diet, and engaging in regular exercise, or by taking drugs like statins, angiotensin-converting enzyme inhibitors, or angiotensin receptor blockers.

Each person with AF has unique characteristics, including age, symptoms, type and duration of AF, risk of stroke, and co-occurring medical disorders, which determine the optimal course of treatment. For AF to be managed safely and efficiently, it is crucial to see a doctor and heed their advice.

Step 10: Eat a balanced diet

Consuming a range of meals that supply the nutrients your body requires to operate well and maintain health is known as eating a balanced diet. A balanced diet can enhance your mood, vitality, and general well-being in addition to assisting in the prevention or management of chronic conditions including diabetes, heart disease, and stroke.

The 2020–2025 Dietary Guidelines for Americans state that the following food groups ought to be a part of a balanced diet:

Fruits and vegetables: Packed with fiber, vitamins, minerals, and antioxidants, these can help reduce your risk of several ailments. A range of colors and varieties of fruits and vegetables should be included in your daily intake, with at least five portions to be consumed. They can be consumed fresh, frozen, canned, dried, or juiced; just don't add salt or sugar.

Whole grains: They contain some protein, fiber, and carbohydrates. They can also help control your cholesterol and blood sugar levels. Choose goods with whole grains as the primary ingredient, and aim to consume half of your grains as whole grains. Oats, brown rice, quinoa, barley, and whole wheat pasta or bread are a few types of whole grains.

Foods high in protein can help build and repair your muscles, bones, and tissues. They are also good sources of iron, zinc, and other nutrients. Eat a range of foods high in protein, such as fish, poultry, beans, lentils, nuts, seeds, eggs, and lean meat; also, cut back on processed meats like ham, bacon, and sausage.

Dairy products or dairy substitutes: They can help strengthen your bones and teeth and are good sources of calcium, protein, and other nutrients. Milk, yogurt, cheese, and soy products are examples of dairy or dairy substitutes that you should consume daily. Opt for low-fat or fat-free varieties. Good fats and oils: They contain unsaturated fats that can protect your heart and brain, increase HDL (good) cholesterol, and lower LDL (bad) cholesterol. Limit your intake of saturated and trans fats, which are found in butter, cream, cheese, coconut oil, palm oil, and baked or fried foods. Instead, choose healthy fats and oils like olive oil, canola oil, sunflower oil, avocado, nuts, seeds, and fatty fish. Along with drinking lots of water, tea, or coffee, you should also cut back on sugary drinks like soda, juice, and sports drinks to maintain a balanced diet. Additionally, you want to stay away from or consume fewer calories from fattening foods, sugary drinks, and salty foods and beverages, including cakes, cookies, candies, chips, fast food, and alcohol. These meals and beverages may include empty calories, which denotes that they are low in nutritional content and may cause weight gain, diabetes, and other health issues.

Consuming a well-rounded diet can be effortless and pleasurable if you adhere to a few basic guidelines, like:

Prepare your meals and snacks in advance, and create a shopping list of wholesome items.

Make your food at home and try to utilize whole, fresh, and minimally processed items.

Instead of adding salt, sugar, or sauces to your dish, use herbs, spices, lemon juice, vinegar, or salsa.

Instead of frying or deep-frying, choose healthy cooking techniques like baking, roasting, grilling, steaming, or microwaving.

Place fruits and vegetables on half of your plate, whole grains in the other quarter, and foods high in protein in the remaining quarter. Top off your plate with a portion of dairy or a dairy substitute.

Eat thoughtfully and slowly, paying attention to your body's signals of hunger and fullness. When you are full, not stuffed, stop eating.

Savor your meals and, in moderation, reward yourself with your favorites from time to time.

One of the best methods to look after your health and well-being is to eat a balanced diet. You can eat a balanced diet that satisfies your nutritional requirements and tastes and reap the rewards of a long and happy life by heeding the advice in this article.

Step 11: Reduce salt intake

Limiting your salt intake is a good practice that can help you avoid fluid retention, lower your blood pressure, and lessen your risk of heart disease and stroke. A mineral called salt, or sodium chloride, is necessary for your body to perform several processes, including neuron and muscle function, fluid balance, and muscular contraction. On the other hand, an excessive amount of salt can make your body retain more water, which can raise blood pressure and volume and put stress on your heart and blood vessels.

According to the 2020–2025 Dietary Guidelines for Americans, people should consume no more than 2,300 mg (or around one teaspoon) of salt each day. Nonetheless, the majority of Americans consume more than this, mostly from restaurants and processed foods rather than from the salt shaker. In the American diet, bread, pizza, sandwiches, soups, snacks, cheese, and cured meats are a few prominent sources of salt.

You can cut back on salt by using the following advice:

Examine the Nutrition Facts labels on packaged foods and select those with no added salt or minimal sodium content. Choose the brands and varieties that have the least amount of salt by comparing them.

Make your own food at home with minimally processed, whole, and fresh ingredients. Instead of adding salt to your dish, flavor it with herbs, spices, vinegar, lemon juice, or salsa. Additionally, you can use low-sodium items to make your own marinades, dressings, and sauces.

Ask for nutrition information when dining out, and select dishes with less sodium. Additionally, you might request that the chef cook your meal with minimal or no salt and refrain from putting soy sauce or salt on the table. Limit your consumption of cheese, bacon, pickles, and olives. Opt instead for baked, steamed, or fried dishes. Increase your intake of fruits and vegetables, which are rich in potassium, a mineral that can help lower blood pressure, and naturally low in sodium. They can be eaten frozen, canned, dried, or fresh; stay away from ones that have sugar or salt added. As an alternative to chips, pretzels, or crackers, you can munch on unsalted nuts, seeds, or popcorn.

To aid in the removal of extra salt from your body, drink lots of water. Restrict the amount of alcohol and sugary drinks you consume, as they can raise your blood pressure and your intake of calories. You can also have unsweetened tea or coffee, as well as low-sodium vegetable or tomato juice.

Cutting back on salt can improve your health and wellbeing, both now and in the future. You can decrease your intake of sodium and enhance your cardiovascular health by implementing these suggestions.

Step 12: Increase potassium intake

For your body to perform its many tasks, including maintaining fluid equilibrium, nerve transmission, and muscle contraction, potassium is a necessary mineral and electrolyte. In addition, potassium helps avoid kidney stones, lower blood pressure, and minimize the risk of stroke.

According to the 2020–2025 Dietary Guidelines for Americans, an adult should get 4,700 mg (or around ten medium bananas) of potassium daily. The majority of Americans, however, do not adhere to this advice and might gain from consuming more potassium.

You can eat more foods high in potassium, such as fruits, vegetables, legumes, nuts, seeds, dairy products, and seafood, to improve your intake of the **mineral**. The following are a few foods with the greatest potassium content per serving:

Avocado: The potassium content of one avocado is 975 mg or 21% of the daily value (DV).

Sweet potato: 328 grams or one cup of mashed sweet potatoes has 766 mg of potassium or sixteen percent of the daily value.

Spinach: 540 mg, or 11% of the DV, can be found in one cup (190 grams) of frozen spinach.

White beans: 829 mg, or 18% of the daily value, are found in one cup (179 grams) of cooked white beans.

fish: 534 mg, or 11% of the DV, is found in one 3-ounce (85-gram) cooked fillet of fish.

You can also use potassium chloride-containing salt replacements in place of sodium chloride, but you should speak with your doctor first because some people may need to restrict their potassium consumption due to medical issues or excessive potassium levels. There are numerous advantages to increasing your potassium consumption for your overall health and well-being. You can enhance your body's functions and lower your chance of developing several ailments by increasing your intake of meals high in potassium.

Step 13: Consume more omega-3 fatty acids

Omega-3 fatty acids are a subtype of polyunsaturated fat that offer several health advantages, including the reduction of inflammation, the lowering of blood pressure and triglycerides, the enhancement of mood and cognitive function, and the prevention or treatment of several illnesses, including depression, rheumatoid arthritis, heart disease, and stroke.

Fish and fish oil are the primary sources of omega-3 fatty acids. These fats are found in two major forms: eicosapentaenoic acid (EPA) and docosahexaenoic acid (DHA). These are the best types of omega-3 fatty acids that are good for your health. Additionally, you can obtain omega-3 from plant sources such as alpha-linolenic acid (ALA), found in flaxseeds, chia seeds, walnuts, soybeans, and canola oil. However, ALA is less powerful and requires your body to convert it inefficiently into EPA and DHA. According to the 2020–2025 Dietary Guidelines for Americans, an adult should take in roughly 250 mg of combined EPA and DHA daily, or roughly two servings of fatty fish per week. Salmon, tuna, sardines, mackerel, and herring are a few types of fatty fish that are high in omega-3 fatty acids. If you do not consume enough fish, you can also take fish oil supplements. However, you should speak with your doctor before taking any supplements, as some may mix with other medications or cause negative effects.

You can use these suggestions to increase your intake of omega-3 fatty acids. Increase your intake of fish and seafood, particularly wild or low-mercury options.

You can steam, roast, or broil your fish, but don't overdo the sauce, butter, or salt. To your salads, smoothies, cereal, or baked goods, add walnuts, soybeans, chia seeds, or flaxseeds. Canola or flaxseed oil can also be used for dressings and cooking.

Select omega-3-fortified meals, including cereal, milk, yogurt, eggs, and bread. Look for goods that include both EPA and DHA, not simply ALA, by reading the labels.

Steer clear of foods high in omega-6 fatty acids, like margarine, sunflower, safflower, or corn oil. The advantages of omega-3 fatty acids may be diminished by competition from omega-6 fatty acids. Aim for an omega-6 to omega-3 balanced ratio, ideally 4:1 or less.

Increasing your intake of omega-3 fatty acids can improve your health and well-being in several ways. You may boost your consumption of omega-3 fatty acids and reap the benefits of a well-balanced diet by heeding these guidelines.

Step 14: Drink more green tea

The popular beverage green tea offers numerous health advantages, including lowering blood pressure and cholesterol, increasing mood and brain function, and preventing or treating several ailments, including diabetes, heart disease, and cancer.

Here are some suggestions to help you drink more green tea:

Use hot, but not boiling, water to brew your green tea, then steep it for only one or two minutes. By doing this, you may help keep the tea's antioxidants intact and avoid bitterness.

To prevent interfering with the absorption of iron from food, sip green tea throughout the day, ideally in between meals. Green tea can also be drunk before or after working out to increase fat-burning and metabolism.

To improve the flavor and health benefits of your green tea, add lemon juice, honey, mint, ginger, or other flavorings. Ginger, honey, and mint can help calm your throat and digestive system, while lemon juice helps boost the antioxidants your body can absorb from green tea. Select premium organic green teas like gyokuro, sencha, or matcha, which are lower in pollutants and pesticides and higher in antioxidants. Additionally, you can experiment with other types of green tea, such as white, oolong, or jasmine tea, each of which has a unique flavor and set of health advantages.

Increased use of green tea can improve your health and well-being in a number of ways. You may reap the benefits of green tea and drink more of it if you heed these guidelines.

Step 15: Eat more dark chocolate

In addition to being a tasty treat, dark chocolate has several health advantages. Cocoa solids, which are used to make dark chocolate, are rich in flavanols, which are antioxidants. Flavonols have anti-inflammatory, heart- and brain-protective, and blood-pressure-lowering properties. They can also enhance blood flow.

You can eat more dark chocolate by using the following advice:

Select dark chocolate with at least 70% cocoa solids instead of milk or white chocolate, as the latter will include less sugar and fat and more flavanols.

Since dark chocolate still includes calories and caffeine, consume it in moderation. Try to limit your daily intake to one or two squares, or 10 to 20 grams.

Savor the rich, bitter taste of dark chocolate as a snack or dessert. For a more filling and healthy treat, you can also combine it with nuts, fruits, or yogurt.

Try a variety of dark chocolate flavors and kinds, like sea salt, orange, chile, and mint. Additionally, since various brands and sources of dark chocolate may have distinct flavors and characteristics, you can experiment with them.

There are numerous advantages to eating more dark chocolate for your health and well-being. You may take advantage of the benefits of dark chocolate and eat more of it by following these guidelines.

Step 16: Take aspirin if prescribed

One medication that can be used to treat pain, fever, and inflammation is aspirin. In addition, it can lessen the chance of blood clots, heart attacks, and strokes. Aspirin is not recommended for everyone, as it can have negative effects or interfere with other medications. Before taking an aspirin, keep the following things in mind:

If you are pregnant or nursing, have a stomach ulcer, have an allergy to NSAIDs or aspirin, or have a bleeding issue, you should not use aspirin.

If you suffer from asthma, gout, liver or kidney issues, heart failure, thyroid issues, or a blood ailment, you should speak with your doctor before using aspirin.

As directed by your physician or the label's dose recommendations, you should adhere to them. Take no more than 4 grams of aspirin in 24 hours.

To prevent an upset stomach, take aspirin with food or drink. Extended-release or enteric-coated tablets should not be chewed, crushed, or broken. Before consuming the chewable tablets, chew them. After gently inserting the suppositories into your anus, lie still for fifteen minutes.

If you use any other medications, notably NSAIDs, steroids, anticoagulants, antiplatelets, or diuretics, you should let your doctor know.

If you experience any of the following symptoms: bruises, nosebleeds, black stools; indicators of bleeding (hives, swelling, difficulty breathing); signs of overdose (ringing in the ears, nausea, vomiting, confusion); or any combination of these symptoms, you should stop taking aspirin and get medical help.

For many ailments, aspirin can be a helpful medication, but it's crucial to take it carefully and sensibly. Any questions or worries you may have regarding taking aspirin should always be directed to your physician or pharmacist.

Step 17: Know the signs and symptoms of a stroke

A stroke is a dangerous medical illness that happens when there is an interruption in the blood supply to a portion of the brain, leading to the death of brain cells. A stroke can result in death or severe disability, as well as long-term brain damage. As a result, it's critical to recognize the warning signs and symptoms of a stroke and to get emergency medical assistance if they materialize.

Typical indications and symptoms of a stroke include the following:

Abrupt facial, arm, or leg numbness or weakness, particularly on one side of the

body Abrupt disorientation, difficulty speaking, or trouble comprehending speech
Unexpected vision problems in one or both eyes
Abrupt difficulty walking, lightheadedness, unsteadiness, or lack of coordination
abrupt, intense headache without apparent cause
The abbreviation F.A.S.T. can be used to help identify a stroke. It stands for:
Face: Request a grin from the person. Does the face sag on one side?
Ask the individual to lift both of their arms. Does one arm sag to the side? Or can only one arm be raised?
Speech: Request that the individual repeat a short word. Is the speaker's speech odd or slurred?
Time: Call 911 or emergency medical assistance as soon as possible if you see

any of these symptoms. Keep track of the moment any symptoms start to show up. Do not wait if you believe you or someone else is experiencing a stroke. Dial 911 or seek emergency medical assistance right now. Every minute matters. The less brain damage and disability that a stroke can cause, the earlier it is treated.

Step 18: Call 911 immediately if you suspect a stroke

If you think someone may be having a stroke, you should call 911 right away to preserve their life and avoid irreversible brain damage. When a portion of the brain's blood supply is cut off, brain cells die, and a stroke happens. The less brain damage and disability that a stroke can cause, the earlier it is treated.

Typical indications and symptoms of a stroke include the following:

Abrupt facial, arm, or leg numbness or weakness, particularly on one side of the body Abrupt disorientation, difficulty speaking, or trouble comprehending speech

Unexpected vision problems in one or both eyes

Abrupt difficulty walking, lightheadedness, unsteadiness, or lack of coordination

abrupt, intense headache without apparent cause

The abbreviation F.A.S.T. can be used to help identify a stroke. It stands for:
Face: Request a grin from the person. Does the face sag on one side?
Ask the individual to lift both of their arms. Does one arm sag to the side? Or can only one arm be raised?
Speech: Request that the individual repeat a short word. Is the speaker's speech odd or slurred?
Time: Call 911 or emergency medical assistance as soon as possible if you see any of these symptoms. Keep track of the moment any symptoms start to show up. When you dial 911, you will speak with a dispatcher who is qualified to pose particular questions to assist emergency medical technicians (EMTs) in locating the patient and determining the severity of their condition. As soon as they can, the EMTs will respond and offer life-saving measures like oxygen, medicine, or CPR. Additionally, they will take the

patient to the closest hospital—such as a comprehensive stroke center—that offers expert stroke care.

If you think someone is having a stroke, the greatest thing you can do for them or yourself is to call 911 right away. Every minute matters. Do not hesitate. Neither you nor the patient should drive to the hospital. Don't hold off until the symptoms subside. Act fast and dial 911.

Step 19: Follow your doctor's advice after a stroke

A stroke is a dangerous medical illness that develops when there is an interruption in the blood supply to a portion of the brain. It can impair several brain processes, including movement, speech, memory, and vision, and result in long-term brain damage. For this reason, it's critical to heed your doctor's advice following a stroke to enhance your recovery and avoid more issues.

Doctors frequently advise stroke sufferers to undertake the following:

Develop a strategy with your physician to reduce your chance of experiencing another stroke. This could entail increasing your level of physical activity, giving up smoking, and controlling your blood pressure, cholesterol, and blood sugar.

As soon as your healthcare team gives you the all-clear, begin your customized rehabilitation program. Early recovery is important. Though recovery can take years, the first few months following a stroke are when many recover the fastest. Take your medications as directed by your doctor. Certain drugs can reduce blood pressure, stop blood clots, or manage other health issues that raise your risk of stroke. Recognize the intended use and potential negative effects of each medicine.

Inquire and look for assistance. After a stroke, it can occasionally be challenging to know what questions to ask your doctor, particularly if you're experiencing neural fatigue and brain fog. Take a list of questions with you to your next doctor's appointment, or use it as a guide. You can print it off. Additionally, look for a support group of individuals who have experienced similar circumstances locally or virtually. They can provide you with coping mechanisms, sensible counsel, and emotional support.

Ensure your emotional well-being. It can be a frightening and stressful experience to have a stroke. It may have an impact on your emotions, mood, and self-worth. You might experience anxiety, anger, frustration, or depression. Although these emotions are common, they may hinder your recuperation. If you require assistance, speak with your physician or a mental health specialist. To help you cope and enhance your quality of life, there are therapies and treatments available.

Remain hopeful and patient. After a stroke, recovery is a difficult and drawn-out process. Sometimes it can be demoralizing and infuriating. But persevere and never give up. Honor your accomplishments, no matter how modest. Consider your strengths rather than your weaknesses. Recall that you are not by yourself. Numerous individuals genuinely care about you and wish to assist you. After a stroke, you can overcome the obstacles and lead a full life with time, effort, and support.

Step 20: Join a stroke support group

One helpful strategy for overcoming the difficulties and adjustments that follow a stroke is to become a member of a support group. A gathering of people who have had a stroke or are providing care for someone who has is known as a stroke support group. They get together regularly to exchange knowledge, encourage one another emotionally, tell their tales, and learn from one another. Among the advantages of being a member of a stroke support group are: You can establish a connection with others who can empathize with you and provide support.

You can get knowledge from the experiences and perceptions of those who have gone through comparable struggles and triumphed over comparable challenges.

After a stroke, you can acquire helpful guidance and pointers on managing your recuperation, rehabilitation, and day-to-day activities.

You get access to useful tools and data regarding stroke treatments, therapies, and prevention.

It is possible to lessen the emotions of melancholy, loneliness, and isolation by interacting with people and forming new acquaintances.

By sharing your successes and advancements with others, you can boost your drive, self-worth, and confidence.

Use the American Stroke Association's Stroke Support Group Finder to locate a stroke support group in your area. For recommendations, you can also speak with your physician, nurse, social worker, or therapist. As an alternative, you can engage with other stroke survivors and caregivers worldwide by joining an online forum or support group.

Joining a stroke support group, whether in person or virtually, can help you gain the understanding, hope, and support that each other in the group can offer. You can learn that you are not alone and that you can lead a happy life after a stroke by joining a support group for stroke victims.

Conclusion

A stroke is a dangerous medical disorder that can affect your body and brain permanently. It need not, however, define your existence. You can take action by heeding the instructions in this book to either prevent a stroke or recover from one.

Controlling your risk factors, which include obesity, alcohol and cigarette use, high blood pressure, high blood sugar, and high cholesterol, is the first step. These elements raise your risk of stroke by causing damage to your blood vessels. You can reduce your risk and enhance your general health by adopting healthy lifestyle choices, including eating a balanced diet, exercising frequently, getting adequate sleep, and giving up smoking.

Understanding the warning signs and symptoms of a stroke, such as abrupt weakness, numbness, disorientation, difficulty speaking, visual issues, or excruciating headaches, is the second stage. Please dial 911 right away if you observe any of these symptoms in yourself or another person. Your chances of surviving and recovering are improved the sooner you receive medical attention. FAST stands for face drooping, arm weakness, speech difficulty, and time to call 911. Keep this acronym in mind. After a stroke, the third stage is to heed your doctor's advice. To aid in your recovery from the stroke and help you avoid having another one, your doctor will give you medicine and a rehabilitation regimen. Adhere to the instructions for your therapy, and take your medications as prescribed. Together with your family, friends, and medical team, create attainable objectives and monitor your advancement. When you need assistance, ask questions and get it. Joining a support group for stroke victims is the fourth stage. A gathering of people who have had a stroke or are providing care for someone who has is known as a stroke support group. They can provide you with coping mechanisms, sensible counsel, and emotional support. You can establish connections with individuals who can relate to your situation and give you motivation to persevere. Along with accessing priceless resources and information, you may also gain knowledge from their experiences and insights.

After a stroke, you can have a happy life by doing these things. You may enjoy the things that are important to you and overcome the obstacles and adjustments that follow a stroke. Along the way, you can support and encourage those who are traveling the same path by demonstrating your bravery and resiliency. Your stroke does not define you, and you are not alone. You can succeed because you are a survivor.

72

www.ingramcontent.com/pod-product-compliance
Lightning Source LLC
Chambersburg PA
CBHW070802250726
48662CB00004B/1930

* 9 7 9 8 8 7 7 8 9 8 9 5 0 *